THE R.A.G. DIET
: lose weight without dieting

Peter Nuttall B.Sc.

ISBN-13: 978-1542485449
ISBN-10: 1542485444

www.peternuttall.net

Contents

Preface

According to the British Heart Foundation, in 2011 the percentage of the UK's population who were overweight had increased by 50% since 2001. There are many reasons why a healthy person can become overweight but the simplest and easiest to control is that of choice; in short, what manner an individual chooses to deal with their hunger and how they fit meals into their daily routines.

The relative low cost and ease of access to foods which are high in refined sugar, saturated fat and salt can lead to a pattern of snacking on unhealthy foods and, because of the body's primitive 'pleasure response' to these tasty foods, can lead to craving these foods even when you aren't hungry. Depending on your lifestyle, if you're on your way somewhere important and you feel hungry, it's easy to call into a local shop and buy a chocolate bar or a packet of crisps. You may decide that chocolate is too unhealthy and opt for a pasty or a pie from the newsagents (which was cooked a few days ago, injected with preservatives and then wrapped in plastic and transported several hundred miles), or perhaps a chicken and bacon sandwich in white bread smothered in mayonnaise? The issue when you're trying to eat well is trying to find a shop that can sell you something filling and healthy off the shelf. It seems at times that nature made everything that is bad for you taste heavenly and everything that is good for you taste like cardboard but there are ways of reducing the amount of fat and 'bad sugar' in your diet whilst ensuring the foods you are eating are still tasty. Eating healthily whilst enjoying what you eat is the key to changing your attitude to food.

A diet is a regime, a quick fix, a program which can work for a short while but is not sustainable. Once the diet is broken, old habits creep back in and the weight begins to increase once more until you catch sight of yourself in the mirror and decide that the chocolate éclair you're currently munching on will be your last whilst saying, "I'll start my diet tomorrow". If you've uttered that sentence more than twice in the last few weeks then this is the book for you. Weight loss can feel like a distant unachievable dream for a lot of people who seem to be on an endless treadmill of different fad diets, abstinence, hunger and unhappiness; but it doesn't have to be that way. 'The R.A.G. diet' will explain how to lose weight slowly, healthily but most importantly of all, sustainably. All of the advice in this book relates to changing your lifestyle and diet for the better; however, if you are in any way unsure about the suggested changes, are currently taking medication or undergoing any other treatment for a medical condition, make sure you speak to your GP beforehand.

The key to the R.A.G. diet working is that you don't cut out the foods you enjoy and look forward to. They're all still allowed as part of your new eating system.

Introduction to the problem with diets

You're probably reading this because you've tried several diets and none of them have worked for you or they *have* worked but they were extremely difficult and once you got down to your target weight and the diet finished, the pounds slowly crept back on until you were back to the weight you were pre-diet within six months.

The problem with a diet is that it is a set of instructions that you must follow regardless of your personal tastes or lifestyle. A diet that makes you to eat a certain type of soup three times a day is impractical if you don't have access to a pan and hob or a microwave three times a day. A diet that tells you to cut out carbohydrate for any length of time isn't going to allow your body to function correctly and therefore can be dangerous. A diet that suggests you eat fish three times a day isn't going to last long if you hate both the taste and the smell of fish. A diet is not sustainable; it can help you to lose weight but it is sometimes demoralising, upsets your sense of wellbeing and happiness and once it's done the job, what then? Back to Pizza every night?

Through all the advice this book has to offer, the key word is change. The way to lose weight healthily and to keep the weight off is to change your attitude to food and your attitude to your health for life. A diet has a beginning (usually a Monday or New Year's Day) and always has an end (a blow-out of sausage rolls, curry and chocolate). The best way to lose weight and to start eating healthily is not to go on a diet at all but to plan what and when you eat around your lifestyle, in effect, making a change you can sustain in the long term so that when people see that you've lost weight you can answer the question "How long have you been on a diet?" with "I'm not *on* a diet".

Before you can be fully on board with the idea of changing your lifestyle and your eating habits you need to have had that 'watershed' moment. That seminal moment when you realised you *had* to do something; when you caught sight of yourself in the mirror of the changing rooms in a clothes shop when you couldn't get your new jeans fastened or the moment you realised you couldn't reach to tie your shoes. It's likely a moment of such magnitude has already happened to you but if it hasn't then you will find it more difficult to muster the will-power to maintain the changes you need to lose weight, feel healthier and happier. If you have had a moment like this however, you need to keep that moment in your mind throughout the initial period of change as there is nothing more motivational.

When diets don't work, some people believe that not eating at all will help them to lose weight. Not only is this dangerous and incredibly unhealthy but once you start eating again, you can end up gaining more weight than you would have beforehand. If you don't eat enough food then your body will eventually be tricked into thinking it needs to store energy for some kind of emergency (in effect, ignoring your fat cells). In its search for an energy source, your body starts to use the only thing available – protein. Humans can't store protein so the body has to get protein wherever it finds it; usually that which is currently performing some kind of structural function. As protein is an essential component of blood, organs and muscle (including cardiac muscle) you can understand why it's a bad idea to allow your body to reach a state where it starts using your own organs and tissues as food. Also, if there is a drop in the amount of carbohydrate in the diet, the body will derive energy from chemicals called ketone bodies. High quantities of ketone bodies can cause the pH of the blood to decrease and become acidic – a state which can occur in untreated Type 1 Diabetes mellitus. The kidneys will attempt to get rid of the ketone bodies by 'flushing them out', which could in turn lead to dehydration.

A fad diet is not the answer.

What is food and why do we need it?

Before we can change how, what and when we eat, we need to understand a little bit more about what food is and what our bodies use it for.

Hunger

Hunger, crudely, is the absence of nutritional components such as carbohydrates and proteins in the blood stream. Hunger is not linked to the contents of the stomach. If you have sufficient nutritional material in your bloodstream and your stomach is empty, you will not feel hungry. When we feel hungry, we feel our stomachs rumbling and doing all kinds of weird things; this is because the lack of essential nutrition in the blood triggers a response in the brain which in turn increases the activity of the stomach and intestines (as these are the places where we extract the essential components of the food we eat). This is why sometimes directly after eating, we can feel even hungrier as the stomach and intestines are receiving messages from the brain to increase their activity to get nutrition into the blood stream as quickly as possible.

Carbohydrate

Food is fuel and is essential to ensuring the body functions correctly. Some diets warn about the dangers of carbohydrate to weight-loss but this couldn't be further from the truth.

Carbohydrate is an essential component in a healthy diet, as are proteins and fats as these are the three components of food which give us energy. Whether you eat fruit, pasta or bread, the carbohydrate in them is treated in the same way by your digestive system. It is broken down where possible, into glucose which then enters the blood stream and is used as an energy source. Carbohydrates have around four calories per gram whereas fat has nine calories per gram. The energy provided by carbohydrates is easier for the body to access than that of fat and as such, are the first nutritional components the body uses.

Any food that tastes sweet such as fruit and syrup is likely to contain high levels of simple carbohydrates, as does white bread, cakes, dairy products and confectionary. Simple carbohydrates are basic sugar molecules which are quickly and easily absorbed into the blood stream and as such, cause rapid changes in blood sugar levels. Insulin controls the uptake of glucose by the body cells that need it. Lots of blood sugar will result in lots of insulin. This increase in insulin will quickly lower the level of blood sugar and quickly lead to hunger, prompting you to have another cake. Any excess sugar that is not taken up into body cells is converted into glycogen and stored in the liver as an energy reserve and the rest is converted into fat and stored. So, as you can see, overeating foods that contain simple sugars can lead to obesity because there is no control on the amount of simple sugars absorbed into the bloodstream and any excess will be converted into fat.

Eating more complex carbohydrates which are found in foods such as bananas, beans, oats, potatoes and wholemeal flour can provide the body with a slower but more sustained release of energy. This slow uptake into the blood means less insulin is needed and as such, there is a much less dramatic fall in blood sugar. Because the sugar is being taken up into the bloodstream much more slowly and for a longer time, you should feel less hungry between meals with the added bonus of less glucose in the bloodstream which could potentially be converted into fat.

Protein

Protein is a complex molecule, much more complex than Carbohydrate. It's made up of individual chemicals called amino acids which are linked together in a chain and takes the body much longer to break down than carbohydrates. There are twenty two standard amino acids, most of which our bodies can manufacture. However, there are some which we cannot produce ourselves and can only enter the body in the foods that we eat. Protein is an essential component of our muscles, organs and blood so it is a vastly important part of our diet. Protein can be found in meat such as chicken and beef, fish such as Tuna and Salmon, milk and eggs. There is a danger of eating too much protein however as the body cannot store it and like excess carbohydrate, can end up being converted into fat.

Fat

Fat is the body's way of storing lots of energy in a small space. A gram of fat has more than twice the energy contained in either a gram of carbohydrate or a gram of protein but fat molecules are complex and release their energy more slowly than simple carbohydrates. Fat is just as important in our diets as any other nutritional component but it is important to understand what the different types of fat are, which are essential and which are bad for us.

Mono-unsaturated and poly-unsaturated
Unsaturated fat, which can be found in olive oil, rapeseed oil, oily fish, sesame seeds and hazelnuts is generally a liquid at room temperature. It contains essential fatty acids which cannot be manufactured by the body and fat-soluble vitamins such as vitamin E. It is believed that mono-unsaturated fat can help to lower high levels of blood cholesterol which can lead to heart disease. Omega-3 is another essential fat which helps to keep the blood healthy.

Saturated
Saturated fat found in butter, cheese, whole milk and pastries is a generally a solid at room temperature. These fats are likely to increase blood cholesterol, increase the risk of heart disease and have even been linked to certain types of cancer.

Trans-fats
Trans-fats are rarely found in nature and were generally only consumed through the milk and fat of ruminants such as cows or sheep. They are not essential fatty acids and are not thought to have any benefit to human health. They increase levels of 'bad' cholesterol and also lower the levels of 'good' cholesterol which can lead to coronary heart disease. Because of this, trans-fats should be avoided in the diet altogether. They are sadly prominent in the western

diet due to their use in the processed food industry. They are used in the production of fast food (fish, chicken and chips especially are deep-fried in hydrogenated oils which contain trans-fats), snack food (boxed cakes and biscuits sold in supermarkets and even reduced-fat crisps can have trans-fats) and baked goods (such as pies, sausage rolls, pasties, cookies and cakes).

Minerals

Dietary minerals are chemical elements needed by the body to perform essential biological tasks such as the production of hydrochloric acid in the stomach or hormones such as thyroxine. Essential minerals include calcium (found in milk), chlorine (found in salt) and iron (found in red meat and eggs). A deficiency in a dietary mineral such as zinc can lead to hair loss and acne while a deficiency in iron can lead to a weakened immune system.

Vitamins

Vitamins are chemical compounds that are either water or fat soluble and are required for the healthy maintenance of organs and tissues. Humans can manufacture some vitamins but most must be obtained from the food that we eat. Vitamins are not stored in the body in great amounts and so must be eaten daily to maintain a healthy supply. Many vitamins have multiple functions and although they are essential to health, it is possible to overdose as well as experience a vitamin deficiency. Too little Vitamin C for example can lead to scurvy but too much vitamin B_3 can lead to liver damage. It is important therefore to maintain a healthy balanced diet that contains a variety of different food groups. Vitamin A is found in Carrots, Vitamin C in citrus fruits and Vitamins E and K in green vegetables.

Water

Water is another essential part of a healthy diet. It is used by the body to help excrete waste products and regulate body temperature among many other functions. In nutrition, it aids digestion and can increase your metabolic rate. Sometimes, when you feel peckish you might actually be craving water, not food. Drinking a glass of water can help to reduce that 'between-meals' hungry feeling. In my experience as a sports therapist, I have treated sportspeople who have complained of sore joints towards the end of a period of exercise. In a healthy active person, this can almost always be attributed to not drinking enough fluids during the workout. Not drinking enough water can also lead to the build-up of toxins in the blood; as the body is attempting to retain water, the kidneys cannot filter out urea, ammonia and other harmful substances.

In females, water can be retained by the body just before the menstrual cycle begins. When monitoring weight as part of a weight-loss program, it can be observed that 'I haven't lost anything this week' as it is possible to gain as much as five pounds through the water that has been retained. This water is lost once more when menstruation ceases.

As well as drinking a glass of water with meals, we can also consume it through fresh fruit and vegetables, milk and hot beverages including tea and coffee. The importance of water in our diet cannot be understated; we can survive for months without food but only a few days without water.

In conclusion

The chemicals your body uses to break down the food you eat into usable building blocks and fuel such as saliva, bile and insulin are themselves made from the foods you eat so it is essential that you provide enough of these proteins, fats, minerals and vitamins to allow the body to function correctly, efficiently and ultimately, be able to convert that excess body fat into energy.

Change for life

The day before the diet starts is the easiest food day as you feel you're free to eat whatever you like guilt-free because tomorrow, you'll start eating healthily. However, tomorrow's enthusiasm soon wanes when hunger starts and you forgot to throw away that bar of chocolate you were keeping in the cupboard for emergencies. The transition from the pig-out on the Sunday and the more conservative intake of food on the Monday is such a significant change that it has an effect on the dieter both physically and mentally.

What and when you eat has to fit into your lifestyle; a slice of toast while getting the kids ready in the morning followed by a cup of coffee when you get to work. Then someone at work suggests that they go on a bacon sandwich run and ask you what you would like; a sausage and onion or a bacon and mushroom roll. Knowing that you shouldn't, the hunger that stabs away at your stomach because of your light breakfast overrides all your desires to be healthy on the first day of your diet. You end up eating the bacon roll, followed by a microwave curry for dinner and because you have to stay late at work and haven't had time to prepare tea, you settle down in front of the TV with a take-away pizza for you, your partner and the kids.

If you're reading that and thinking that won't happen, you can be sure a variant of that tale with happen sooner or later, usually within the first two weeks. Justifing it by saying that you've eaten well for six days in a row is something many dieters do too.

Habits

Bad eating is habitual; it's a cycle which repeats, sometimes day to day or more likely week to week. The eating habits you have developed over time feel almost impossible to break. This is why a diet can be stressful on the mind as well as the body. If you have been eating unhealthily, then you will already be depriving your body of essential nutrients which can cause stress on your physiology, but suddenly switching away from what your body is used to will also bring about major changes in your mood and wellbeing. With all that going on, whatever willpower you had on the Monday morning can be severely tested as early as 3pm on the same Monday afternoon. A change in how you think about food is the answer as it relieves all the pressure you put yourself under when you're on a diet. In social situations for example, when you're out for a meal with friends, scanning the menu for plain chicken and lettuce completely spoils the point of your night out.

Ensuring that you're eating correctly for the rest of the week means you can order roast duck linguini, enjoy your night out and find that you've still lost a pound at the end of the week. You'll also learn that when you've had what you consider to be a 'sinful' meal, you don't have to punish yourself the next day by eating only mange-tout dipped in mineral water. The R.A.G. diet allows you to have one day a week which involves sinful eating. You just need to ensure you're eating correctly for the other six.

Will power is impossible to maintain if the dietary rules you inflict upon yourself are too strict. This becomes more true when you start to make headway in your weight-loss; the rules change and bad habits start to creep back in such as snacking between meals with foods which have low nutritional value and are high in processed and refined ingredients. Only when you've gone through this cycle of dieting and giving up can you fully appreciate the value of a long term change in your attitude to food.

She eats what she wants and never gains weight

It's not uncommon to see people of slender frame eating what seems like nothing but chocolate, crisps and bacon sandwiches. No matter what they eat, they never seem to put on weight. Everyone has a different metabolic rate but if you know someone like this and you feel jealous of their ability to 'eat what they like and not gain weight', take a look at their skin, hair and nails; ask them if they feel sluggish and suffer from chronic heart-burn. You'll find out that their general health suffers because they gauge their food intake by the girth of their waistline; to them, skinny equals healthy. Some of the fat in a person's body is essential. It is found beneath the skin for insulation and around organs for protection. It is healthy therefore to have fat in the body and one cannot gauge health by the amount of visceral fat (the fat in the abdomen) one has. The slim people you see stuffing their faces with chocolate every day may have an excellent Body Mass Index (BMI) but they are putting themselves at risk of other physiological complications such as diabetes due to insulin resistance and raised blood cholesterol which can lead to heart disease. Also, although oxygen is essential to life, it is also a highly reactive element and can form *reactive oxygen species* which react readily with cellular components and cause damage.

Also produced within cells are bodies known as free radicals which can cause damage to DNA and proteins in the body. This DNA damage can lead to mutations and sometimes cancerous cells. Vitamins C and E both act as anti-oxidants and inhibit the action of free radicals in the body. Vitamin C is thought to lower rates of cancer in the mouth and oesophagus because of its anti-oxidant properties and Vitamin E is thought to have a similar effect in protecting against cardiovascular disease by inhibiting the formation of the plaque which blocks the arteries. So, the next time you see your skinny friend shoving chocolate in their face and you look on with jealous eyes, remember that they're putting themselves at great risk not only because of their high sugar and fat intake, but also because of their low intake of essential vitamins and minerals.

Overeating and under eating

Eating is a way of overcoming boredom for some overweight people. The time you spend between dinner at six in the evening and bedtime is filled with television and something to 'keep you going' until bedtime. This pre-sleep snack is a method of preventing yourself from becoming emotionally bored. It could also be because you're used to eating foods which are high in sugar and you're experiencing the 'low' brought about by the natural lowering of the level of sugar in your blood and this evening snack is a way of perking up your mood which will have dipped as your metabolism slows. There are many other emotional states which will lead to overeating too – feeling low or depressed can make you think the only thing that will help you through the day is the thought of a Chinese take-away when you get home. The thought of crisp-breads and a glass of water for tea isn't going to cut it.

Being on a diet, however euphoric the feeling of seeing that lower number the next time you step on the scales, is never enough to temper those dark moods when you're tired, bored, unhappy and hungry. Diets also have a danger of altering your attitude to food to the opposite extreme where you become scared of eating. You almost feel like anything other than a carrot for dinner and you'll be back to square one. This couldn't be further from the truth; you have to eat to lose weight, in fact you have to eat a range of things to lose weight. Later in the book I will make some suggestions for meals you can eat when you change your eating habits which can help towards losing weight; and they will surprise you. The world is full of inviting and tempting culinary sins; a chocolate shop on every corner, bakeries with cream cakes stuffed in the window and coffee shops offering a free shot of syrup and a curl of whipped cream on top of your skinny mocha. The truth is you can still enjoy these things once a week; all you have to do is manage your meals and slowly learn to change your behavioural consumption. The rest of this book will give you everything you need to do just that whilst explaining the easy R.A.G. system.

Stage 1 : Preparing for change

You are about to embark on a change for life which sounds daunting, but if you plan correctly beforehand, you can help smooth the transition from your current lifestyle and eating habits to the new healthier ones. This section of the book will help you to understand what to change and how to change. How to eat healthily while still looking forward to your meals, planning your new weekly eating program, how to stay strong in times of weakness or if you feel like giving up altogether until one day you realise that you've changed and didn't even notice it. If you're changing to lose weight for the long-term then there are some essentials you need to consider. You will also need some simple things to help keep track of your R.A.G., which stands for 'Red, Amber, Green'. More of this below.

Scales

Buy a set of accurate digital scales. They are an essential component in keeping track of your progress in the initial stages. Once you're down to your target weight, weighing yourself weekly will help you to keep on top of any fluctuations which you can address accordingly. Make sure the scales are in the exact same place on your floor each time you use them and use them on a hard flat floor too.

Tape measure

If you are changing in order to lose weight as well as improving your general wellbeing, then you'll need a tape measure. Fat is deposited mainly in the abdomen but can also be deposited under the skin; in females on the waist, hips and buttocks and in males, the chest, abdomen and buttocks. Keeping track of the girth of certain body parts will give you a valuable indication as to how the weight loss is going. You can also track this by trying on certain clothing which used to fit but doesn't any longer. Trying this item of clothing on every few weeks will also help you track your weight lost.

Spreadsheet or notebook

Start a spreadsheet with the date at the start of each row and the columns headed with measurements of the areas you expect to lose weight from. The best areas to measure are the girth of the waist, belly, chest and buttocks. Add another column for your weight, whether in pounds and ounces or Kilograms.

A physical weight

Whether this is a dumbbell or something else you know the exact weight of (could be a bag of sugar or similar) it is an invaluable tool in remaining motivated. If you climb on your scales to find you've only lost ¼ of a pound (4 ounces), it will motivate you to pick this weight up and physically understand how much that is. Healthy weight loss can be around one to one and a half pounds a week – this is around half a kilogram. Find a foodstuff in your home that has '500g' written on the packet and feel the weight. Suddenly that dejected feeling of 'I only lost a pound' turns into 'wow, I lost a whole pound this week'.

Felt tip pens

You will need a green, red and yellow (or orange) pen. This is how you will track your red, green and amber days.

Calendar

Not only will you have to colour in your days to keep track of how many green, red and amber days you've had per week, having an appreciation of both time scale and frequency of habit is a very good motivational tool. Remember, change isn't easy and it will take time to adapt to new eating habits before they become second nature.

Writing your starting weight on the first day of eating healthily will show you just how far you've come in a relatively short time. Eating correctly using the advice in this book can lead to a loss of up to two stone in just three months. This is hugely dependent on your existing Body Mass Index, dietary requirements and general health, but generally speaking, even if you are only three stone overweight, you can see a difference of up to two stone in just twelve weeks.

The weighing habit

Good practice for tracking weight loss is to weigh yourself once a week on the same day and time every week. However, because you can see a change of up to eight ounces or 227 grams from one day to the next (depending on whether you've just eaten or whether you've gotten rid of the last thing you ate yet among other factors) you should weigh yourself at say, 9am on a Saturday morning and then again at 9am on the Sunday morning and take an average. Whatever you do, NEVER weigh yourself on the five days in-between as any gains you see could be down to water-retention or natural fluctuations in body contents and can only have a negative effect on your determination to maintaining the changes you have made.

Exercise plan

If you exercise, you use more calories and if you use more calories than you take in through food then you will have to turn to the fat stored in your body for energy, which in turn makes you lose weight. It is unhealthy not to exercise however as just 30 minutes exercise, three to five times a week not only helps your respiratory and circulatory systems to stay healthy, but can also reduce stress, increase the levels of 'happy hormones' and help you to feel less sluggish and tired. It is important to have an exercise plan such as a thirty minute aerobic circuit and a weekly rota. Exercise is extremely helpful but not wholly necessary for weight loss. By that I mean it's absolutely possible to lose weight without exercising but much easier if you do. If you feel unwell or are unable to exercise for whatever reason, you shouldn't worry about missing one or two sessions as this won't have a great impact on your weight loss for that week.

Prepare for the changes

New foods and new habits will have an effect on your body. Think about the foods you have been eating and compare them to the ones you'll be changing to. Your body is going to have to adjust to different, healthier levels of sugar, fat, protein, minerals and vitamins. It may not have to work so hard to find the things it needs to maintain health. The levels of stomach acid produced will change, as will the levels of bile produced by the liver and stored in the gall bladder. You may find that you never feel bloated any more or that heartburn you used to get all the time has never returned since you changed.

Support mechanism

As you can imagine, the most difficult way to change is on your own. If you are in the same room as someone who is tucking into *your* favourite Chinese take-away while you are eating your roast chicken and steamed vegetables, you'll find it hard to stay focussed. Finding a support mechanism is very important. If not a partner or another member of the family, having a friend or work colleague who is going through the same changes you are can help immeasurably.

You might find that all you talk about is food, what you've eaten that day, how you deal with hunger pangs between meals and how much weight you've lost but you'll probably find the whole period of change very difficult unless you have someone to share it with. You could get the whole family involved – asking your children to come up with ideas for meals and increasing your general health and fitness as a family. Eventually the changes you've made will become your way of life and in time you will forget that you even made a change in the first place, it will all become part of your natural routine.

Recipe book

Try to find a recipe book which is themed around healthy eating. Even better (because it's free) have a look on the website *Pinterest* (uk.pinterest.com) I have included some recipes in this book to help you find new and healthier ways to keep on enjoying the seemingly unhealthy foods you used to eat. Cooking food yourself instead of relying on prepared meals from supermarkets will reduce the amount of processed ingredients, preservatives and other additives you consume.

It is important to plan your meals for the week ahead. Write down what you're having for lunch and tea for the entire week. That way you can buy the ingredients in advance and each day, prepare your meals fresh without coming home from work and wondering what there is in the cupboards and turning to a take away. This will keep you on the straight and narrow.

You will also increase the amount of fresh ingredients you consume; the ones with the essential vitamins and minerals. Flavouring chicken with herbs and spices, roasting it and serving it with steamed vegetables will give you peace of mind that you're consuming all the necessary components you need for a balanced and healthy diet. A good recipe book will also give you a fresh menu of dishes you'd never have thought of previously. Not only will this vary your diet and ensure you're eating correctly, it dispels the myth that you have to have salad for tea and ensures you look forward to meal times.

Once you have these essentials, you need to draw up a simple time-table. Pick a time and day to measure and weigh yourself, pick days and times to exercise and most importantly, plan your meals in advance.

Stage 2 : The Food Map

The food map is another important tool in facilitating how you are going to initiate and maintain the changes you are about to make. If you don't make a food map, then you'll find yourself at the fridge every day, shaking your head and wondering what to have for dinner. The next thing you know, the take-away menu is in your hand and you're halfway through ordering the house special for two.

A food map is a list of all the things you like to eat and all the things you need to eat. You can then start to formulate a list of meals, snacks and drinks that you can feel 'safe' putting on your weekly menu. Stick the list on a notice board or the fridge and when you run out of an ingredient, cross it off and transfer it to your shopping list for next week. This will ensure you never run out of something you'll end up substituting with something you shouldn't. Later in this chapter there is a sample food map; it starts with an example shopping list and following it is a day by day food plan with recipes. Once you are comfortable with your own food map you won't need to make lists but it's always a good idea to plan your meals for the week to lessen the possibility of going to the cupboards and realising there's only one possible meal you can have and you don't fancy it.

Next you need to colour code your food. The R.A.G. diet is simple in its set up but requires you to understand what constitutes a red day, a green day and an amber day. A green day is a day when you've had three healthy meals with no snacking. An amber day is one where you have snacked and a red day is one where you have eaten badly. You are allowed one of the following each week :

1. Six green days and one red day
2. Five green days and two amber days

You should use your common sense when classifying your food. You'll know what you can eat on each of these days after a while but for clarity :

1. Green days will involve three healthy meals, no snacking and no eating at all after 7pm.
2. Amber days are essentially green days with one snack which does not exceed 300 calories (i.e. a chocolate bar, bowl of ice cream, pint of beer etc.)
3. A red day is what you'd expect. It's probably best to only have one 'treat' on this day for the first few months as you're starting to lose the weight but as you move into the secondary stage, as long as you've stuck to the six green day regime, you can eat pretty much whatever you like within reason of course.

Your calendar will have lots of green on it, a smattering of yellow and never more than four red days a month. If you look at your calendar and there's more red than that, it should cause you a deal of reality and set you back on the right path.

Substituting

A great way to start reducing the amount of calories you eat without compromising on the foods you enjoy is to substitute. Swapping what could be deemed as high fat or high calorie foods with ones that contain less fat or calories. Supermarkets have 'nutrition wheels' on products these days and help identify those foods with high calories and fat content easily. Be warned however, check what quantity of the food they are basing their values on. You could pick up a tub of double cream and see that one gram only contains 0.2 grams of saturated fat – which sounds like it can't be bad for you. However, the whole tub is probably 300 grams and therefore you will be consuming 60 grams of saturated fat. This is true of most foods; rarely on the front of the pack do they list the calories or fat content of the entire contents.

Often there will be tiny writing above the 'nutrition wheel' which states 'values based on ¼ of a pack'. With this in mind however, substituting really is as simple as it sounds and here are some examples:

Lean meat

Instead of buying streaky bacon or the type that has lots of that white rind attached to it, look for lean cuts. Supermarkets have specific brands these days called things like 'be good to yourself'. Compare the nutritional information on a pack of normal bacon with the 'be good' pack and you'll see how much difference there actually is. Choose pork chops without the fatty rind, lean mince and chicken without skin.

Skimmed milk

Milk has excellent nutritional value but there are huge differences between skimmed and whole milk. A cup of whole milk has 150 calories and 8 grams of fat whereas skimmed milk only has 90 calories and 0.5 grams of fat. The fact that the milk is 'skimmed' doesn't have any effect on its protein, phosphorus, calcium and potassium levels. There is a taste difference of course but once you start using skimmed milk, the benefits soon outweigh the difference in flavour.

Lighter spreads

There are a variety of lower fat butters on the market these days. Some also claim to be able to lower your cholesterol. However, just because it is 'lower' in fat, doesn't mean it's good for you. Used sparingly for those of you who love the taste and can't have toast without it means you are still enjoying your food whilst lowering your overall intake of fats and calories. Remember also to avoid any spread which has trans-fats or hydrogenated oils.

Fluid plant oils

If you're frying your food, make sure you use oils which only contain very low levels of saturated fat. Canola oil is very low in saturated fat, as is olive oil. Never use solid fats or animal fats for cooking. The health benefits of using plant oil over animal fats are huge and massively outweigh any negatives caused by the differences in taste.

Snacks

You probably look to cakes, biscuits and crisps between meals when you feel a bit hungry. Hopefully, when you change what you eat at meal-times, you won't feel hungry between meals. If you do however, try eating fresh fruit such as a banana or an apple, nuts or having a low calorie hot drink such as a flavoured hot chocolate. One of my clients told me of his 'renaissance' moment which involved him looking down at his lunch of 'tuna in full-fat mayonnaise sandwiches in white bread' and realising that he hadn't eaten any vegetables at all for as long as he could remember (except chips). He now eats at least three different fruit or vegetables a day and has lost a significant amount of weight (healthily) in just a few months.

Breakfast

Don't substitute breakfast with a cereal bar. The benefits of having something like porridge, which releases its energy slowly, raises your metabolism, stops you feeling hungry for longer and as a result can improve your moods and concentration levels in the morning, far outweigh the 'quick fix' of a cereal bar. Some cereal bars are high in fat or sugar and some of them are high in both. You should regard them as confectionary rather than cereal and avoid them as a substitute for the first (and most important) meal of the day.

Tortilla wraps and brown bread

Most of us know that brown bread is far healthier than white, but why? In my opinion, it is one of the most important changes you can make if all you have ever eaten is white bread. There is such a taste difference between white and wholemeal that it can be difficult to change, but once you've switched and gotten used to the new flavour you will never look back. Try changing to one of those 'half and half' loaves first and then maybe to rye bread to make the transition easier. Whole-wheat bread contains vitamin E, vitamin B, Iron, folic acid and copper. The main source of nutrition in wholemeal bread comes from the bran and the germ which is completely removed in the production of white bread. Some bread manufacturers replace elements such as fibre and vitamin B3 which are stripped in the production of the wheat flour. Therefore it's better to eat the wholegrain where these elements occur naturally than have them stripped out and replaced artificially. After suggesting to many of my clients over the years that they switch to wholemeal bread, most have said they had never felt bloated since changing and one, who used to experience chronic heartburn most days has never had heartburn since.

Low fat cheese

Cheese isn't wholly bad as a foodstuff but lots of people love it and find themselves sprinkling it liberally on pizzas and jacket potatoes. It is high in protein, calcium and phosphorus but it is worth remembering that a lot of cheeses are also high in saturated fat. Taking in less calories and fat in your new lifestyle could mean simply cutting down on the amount of cheese you eat but there are now brands of cheese on the market that are lower in calories and fat without compromising too much on taste and texture. Again, it will be a case of adapting to the taste of the new cheese and understanding the different characteristics of the new cheese in your cooking but once you do, it will be an important and positive change to make if you love cheese and can't do without it. Another way to cut down on the amount you consume is to use mature cheese. This has a much stronger flavour and means you won't need to use as much.

Low fat sausages

It might surprise you to see how low in fat certain brands of sausages are. There is a supermarket which sells sausages which encourage you to 'be good' and at only 2.6g of fat per 100g, it's another way of dramatically reducing your fat intake whilst maintaining your love affair with certain purported bad foods.

Grill and bake

Even when using plant oils to fry your food, it's going to increase the amount of fat in your diet and choosing to grill or bake your food instead will give you more leeway if you're finding it difficult to compromise in other areas. If you like chicken curry for example, grilling or baking your chicken instead of frying it, then slicing it and adding it to the sauce is an excellent way of reducing your fat intake. Steaming vegetables is a great way of ensuring none of their vitamins and minerals are lost the way they can be if you boil them.

There are many more examples, so take a look at your food map and tick the foods you know to be less healthy and see if you can find alternatives on the supermarket shelves. This could be the difference between an amber day and a green day, leaving a day of the week free for your red day! Another excellent substitution method to employ is to make meals from scratch. It will take more planning than throwing a frozen meal in the microwave but by making meals with fresh ingredients from scratch you can be sure you are not consuming all the refined ingredients which will have a detrimental effect on your weight loss and ultimately your lifestyle.

There is a recipe in the next section for homemade beef burgers. You'd think in order to eat healthy, beef burgers would be off the menu completely but when you hand-make them with lean mince and fresh diced onions you'll begin to understand how you can start making those changes you need for a healthier lifestyle without the need to deprive yourself of the food you enjoy.

Example shopping list and weekly eating plan

Below is the shopping list which provides all of the items you need for the food map which follows. This is just an example of the type of thing you should do, exchanging foods and meals in the examples with your own favourites. Be aware however that your breakfasts should include slow-energy-release foods to help maintain your hunger and increase metabolism in the morning, helping you to lose weight and feel more awake.

You must consume something from every food group every day:

- Carbohydrates (potatoes, rice, pasta, wholemeal bread, fruit and vegetables)
- Protein (meat, fish, poultry, eggs, beans and dairy products)
- Fat (dairy products, red meat, oily fish and nuts)
- Fibre (cereal, wholemeal bread and vegetables)
- Minerals and vitamins (fruit, vegetables, milk and eggs)

The suggestions in brackets are by no means exhaustive; once you have made your initial food map and decided on a daily eating pattern, make sure all six of the above food groups are present each day. It is good practice to pin your weekly eating plan on a notice board or the fridge so you get into the habit of looking at the next day's meals and realising that you need to 'defrost the chicken' or 'marinade the pork chops'. There's nothing more frustrating when you've just started your new plan when you look at your list and realise that the fish you'd planned to have for dinner that evening is still in the freezer three minutes before you were due to put it in the oven.

The plan below is, in general, the plan that I drew up for one of my clients. It enabled him to drop from seventeen stone to just under fourteen stone in sixteen weeks. Eating out (having lasagne or fish and chips in a restaurant) and having a 'treat' (such as a scoop of ice cream at the pictures) or still being able to fuel his take-away habit by having one take-away a week (i.e. a red day) ensured he didn't get bored with his new program and he now has a completely different leaner and healthier lifestyle.

Shopping list

Bran flakes
Orange juice
Apple juice
4 x bananas
1 x pack of sweet chilli chicken slices
1 x pack of tikka chicken slices
2 x large yellow peppers
1 x large cucumber
1 x punnet chestnut mushrooms
1 x bag frozen roasting parsnips
2 x 250g lean mince
1 x iceberg lettuce
1 x bag frozen peas
1 x bag frozen sweetcorn
1 x bag of new potatoes
1 x lemon sole fillet
1 x pack smoked lean ham
Lightly salted popcorn
2 x Eggs
Tomatoes
Strawberries
Black grapes
Onion
Oregano
Parsley
Salt
Lo-calorie flavoured hot chocolate
Ground black pepper
Breadcrumbs
Wholemeal buns
Porridge
Dried mango
Vegetable soup
Wholemeal bread
Pack of three peppers (red yellow green)
English mustard
2 x microwave rice
Low-calorie tikka sauce

Chicken breasts x4
Thyme
Wholemeal spaghetti
Broccoli
Sesame seeds
125ml single cream
Parmesan
Jar of pickled beetroot
Packet of carrot batons
8 x spring onions
Coriander
250g minced turkey
Fresh root ginger
Bottle of light soy sauce
Bottle of sesame oil
Jar of mint sauce
Bottle of olive oil
Powdered garlic or 1 x garlic bulb
1 x Lemon
Beef stock
Chilli Powder
200g canned kidney beans
Tomato puree
Lean bacon medallions

Monday (Green Day)

Breakfast
Bran Flakes[1]
Orange juice[2]

Mid-morning
Banana[3]

Lunch
Salad[4] (50g chilli chicken slices[5], 1 sliced yellow pepper, ¼ large cucumber (sliced), 4 sliced chestnut mushrooms, chopped iceberg lettuce, 100g fresh strawberries[6])

Dinner
Home-made burgers with roasted parsnips (See below for recipe)

Supper (optional)
Hot drink[7]

[1] Bran flakes provide a large dose of fibre which not only stops you feeling hungry longer but keeps things moving in the colon and keeps you regular. It can be an acquired taste so stick with it., it's worth it.
[2] Any small glass of fresh fruit juice will do
[3] You don't need the banana if you don't feel hungry but it's a great way of managing any hunger you feel between breakfast and lunch as it is full of slow-energy release complex carbohydrates.
[4] Salads are perceived to be boring but by choosing sweet, juicy salad vegetables, it doesn't have to be.
[5] Look in your local supermarket for the different types of cooked poultry and meats you can buy to add to your salad in order to make it tastier and add that much needed protein.
[6] Adding fruit to a salad that contains meat isn't as crazy as it sounds. If you get the right combination (pineapple and ham for example) it can boost the palatability of a salad you'd otherwise find boring.
[7] Avoid the various malted drinks on the market; any hot drink that you enjoy will have a positive psychological effect and help you sleep better. Try a low calorie flavoured hot chocolate drink such as 'options'.

Home-made burgers with roasted parsnips

Ingredients (serves 2)
250g lean mince
Half an onion (diced)
1 teaspoon of oregano
1 teaspoon of parsley
¼ teaspoon of salt
1 teaspoon of pepper
½ cup of breadcrumbs
1 small egg
2 x Soft wholemeal buns
Lettuce to garnish
75g frozen or fresh roasting parsnips

Method

1. Cover the parsnips with pepper and thyme and place them in the oven for 25 minutes on 190 degrees.
2. Add the mince, onions, salt, pepper, oregano, parsley and egg into a mixing bowl.
3. Mix it all together with your hands. (Mix just enough to combine all the ingredients, as over-mixing will spoil the texture of the burger)
4. Depending on your taste, divide the mince into four for smaller burgers or two for larger ones.
5. Pat the mince into pattie shapes (Squeezing tightly to ensure it is packed tightly and won't fall apart in the cooking process) and grill for around 20 minutes turning occasionally.
6. To avoid over cooking use the "drop hinge" on your bench-top grill or ensure you turn the burgers frequently if you're using a conventional grill.
7. Once cooked, add to the bun, garnish with lettuce and serve up with the roasted parsnips.

Compare this to a burger you'd buy in a fast food restaurant and if you're thinking it just doesn't taste the same, that's because this one doesn't contain those chemicals you don't need.

Tuesday (Green day)

Breakfast
Bran Flakes
Orange juice

Mid-morning
Banana

Lunch
50g tikka chicken slices, 1 sliced yellow pepper, ¼ large cucumber (sliced), 4 sliced chestnut mushrooms, chopped iceberg lettuce, 100g fresh black grapes

Dinner
Sesame Turkey meatballs (see below for recipe).

Supper (Optional)
Hot drink

Sesame Turkey meatballs with minted peas and Sweetcorn

Ingredients (serves 2)
2 spring onions
10g Coriander (pre-chopped)
250g minced turkey (or other minced poultry)
5 teaspoons of sesame seeds
Fresh root ginger
2 teaspoons light soy sauce
2 tablespoons sesame oil
1 egg white
Frozen sweetcorn
Frozen Peas
Two table spoons mint sauce

Method
1. Place the minced Turkey into a mixing bowl
2. Chop spring onions and add to the bowl with the Turkey.
3. Add the coriander, sesame seeds, soy sauce, ginger and egg white to the mixture.
4. Mush the mixture together for thirty seconds until fully mixed together.
5. Divide the mixture into ten small meatball shapes and place on a plate.
6. Chill in the fridge for twenty to thirty minutes. This will prevent them falling apart in the frying process.
7. Heat the peas and sweetcorn in separate pans of water.
8. Heat the sesame oil in a frying pan and add the meatballs. Turn the meatballs frequently to ensure they are cooked evenly on all sides and right through to the middle.
9. Once the meatballs are almost ready, drain the sweetcorn and peas. Using a tablespoon, drizzle the mint sauce over the peas and mix thoroughly.
10. Serve and enjoy

The best thing about this recipe is adjusting the ingredients to suit your tastes. I personally prefer to use more ginger and soy sauce. Also check out the benefits of using both sesame oil and sesame seeds.

Wednesday (Green day)

Breakfast
Porridge
Apple juice

Mid-morning
100g dried mango

Lunch
Vegetable soup with two slices of whole-meal bread

Dinner
Lemon Sole with roast mushrooms and peppers

Lemon Sole with roasted mushrooms and peppers

Ingredients (serves 1)

1 x lemon sole fillet
1 x green pepper
1 x red pepper
3 x sliced chestnut mushrooms
3 x teaspoons of olive oil
2 x tablespoons of thyme
1 x teaspoon of freshly chopped or powdered garlic
1 x lemon
50g of breadcrumbs

Method

1. Pre-heat the oven to 190°C.
2. Chop the peppers and mushrooms and place them into a large sandwich bag.
3. Add the olive oil to the bag, tie the top and shake until the peppers and mushrooms are fully coated.
4. Place the peppers and mushrooms on a baking tray and space them out.
5. Place the lemon sole on a baking tray and brush with olive oil. Squeeze the lemon onto the fish and then sprinkle lightly with breadcrumbs.
6. Sprinkle the thyme over the peppers, mushrooms and fish.
7. Sprinkle the garlic over the mushrooms only.
8. Place in the oven for 25 minutes.

The beauty of this dish is in the flavours you add to the peppers and mushrooms. You could roast them without adding garlic and thyme, using low fat vinaigrette to dress them once cooked.

Thursday (Green day)

Breakfast
Porridge
Glass of Apple Juice

Mid-morning
Mocha with skimmed-milk

Lunch
Lean smoked ham and English mustard sandwiches made with whole-meal bread.

Dinner
Chicken Curry (See below for recipe)

Chicken curry

Ingredients (serves 2)

    1 x Packet of microwave rice
    1 x Jar of low calorie Tikka Sauce
    2 x Chicken breasts
    1 x Teaspoon Thyme
    ¼ Teaspoon of salt
    1 x Teaspoon of pepper

Method

1. Pre-heat oven to 190 degrees
2. Place two chicken breasts on baking tray and cover with thyme, salt & pepper.
3. Place the chicken in the oven for 25 minutes.
4. Pour the jar of Tikka Sauce to a pan and warm 5 minutes before the chicken is ready.
5. When chicken is ready cut into strips and add to the sauce. Heat for one minute.
6. Place naan breads in the oven for 3 minutes to warm.
7. Cook the rice as instructed on the packet.
8. Once the rice is cooked, dish up!

There are some tasty low calorie curry sauces on the market – weight watchers do a tasty tikka sauce but shop around and be sure to check the calorie and fat content of the jar you choose. You can also buy 'be good to yourself' type naan breads which are small, tasty and allow you to enjoy your meal with a much lower calorie content without compromising on taste.

Friday

Breakfast
Bran Flakes

Mid-morning
Banana

Lunch
100g flavoured cooked poultry, cucumber, 1 yellow pepper (sliced), five slices of pickled beetroot, carrot batons, iceberg lettuce.

Dinner
Chilli con carne

Chilli con carne

Ingredients (Serves 2)

2 x tablespoons olive oil
1 x chopped onion
1 x diced red pepper
1 x crushed garlic clove or 1 tsp of powdered garlic
250g lean minced beef
275ml beef stock
1 x teaspoon chilli powder
200g canned kidney beans
200g chopped tomatoes
1 x tablespoon tomato puree
1 x sprinkle of salt and pepper
125g brown long-grain rice

Method

1. Gently heat the oil in a pan then add the red pepper and the onions. Stir for 3 minutes until gently fried.
2. Add the garlic and stir for a further minute.
3. Add the meat and increase the heat to the pan slightly.
4. Stir and separate the meat until it turns brown. Add the chilli powder, tomatoes, tomato puree, beans, salt, pepper and the beef stock.
5. Stir the mixture whilst bringing it to the boil. Cover the pan and reduce the heat. Simmer for about forty minutes, stirring every five to ten minutes to ensure the mixture doesn't stick to the base of the pan.
6. Boil the rice ten minutes before the chilli con carne is cooked or use microwavable rice which is quicker, easier and equally as tasty.
7. Place half of the rice on each of two plates then add a few spoons of the chilli con carne to the top of the rice.
8. Enjoy.

Saturday (Green Day)

Breakfast
Bran flakes

Lunch
Eat out[1]

Dinner
Pasta Carbonara followed by banana ice cream[2]

[1]*You are allowed to eat out, even when you're in the first few weeks of your new way of eating. There are many restaurants now that put the calories of a meal on the menu. Just remember what we've covered in the rest of this book and choose the healthiest options. Fajitas are good; just leave the sour cream and cheese. Cajun chicken with salad is good too but just remember what tastes great without being too high in fat. Try only eating half the fries too and choose a low calorie dip to make them taste amazing.*

[2]*Slice a banana and place it in the freezer. When you take it out an hour later, let it defrost a little and it tastes exactly like banana ice cream!*

Pasta Carbonara

Ingredients (serves 2)

1 x garlic clove or 1 tsp of powdered garlic
Half an onion (diced)
3 x tablespoons of olive oil
5 x rashers of lean smoked bacon medallions
200g wholemeal spaghetti
2 x tablespoons of parmesan
8 x tablespoons of single cream
1 x tablespoons of ground pepper
1 x egg
Chopped Parsley to garnish

Method

1. Bring a pan of water to the boil and add the spaghetti. Turn down to a low heat.
2. Place the oil, chopped garlic and diced onion in a pan on a low heat for five minutes.
3. Chop the bacon into small pieces , add to the pan and simmer.
4. Using a mixing bowl, mix the egg, single cream, parmesan, and pepper together.
5. When the pasta has cooked drain into a colander and then add the pasta to the onion, garlic and bacon . Stir until it is all mixed together.
6. Turn the heat off and add the egg/cream mixture immediately. Toss well and serve with a garnish of parsley

This recipe uses bacon which is very low in fat instead of the usual pancetta, which is extremely high in fat yet still tastes fantastic. Explore low fat cheese options too but don't be afraid of food like this. Even if you have this meal once a week, you'll find that sticking to 3 set meals with healthy snacks, you'll continue to lose weight healthily. Again, play around with the quantities. Add more garlic or more pepper for extra bite.

Sunday (Red day)

Breakfast
Porridge

Lunch
Summer Sunday roast (See recipe below)

Mid-day snack
Lightly salted popcorn

Dinner
Take-away Pizza

Summer Sunday Roast

Ingredients (serves 2)

2 x skinless chicken breasts
50g frozen broccoli
50g frozen peas
100g small potatoes
1 x teaspoon of thyme
Sprinkle of salt and pepper
Gravy

Method

1. Put the potatoes into a pan of boiling water for thirty minutes.
2. Pre-heat the oven to 190 degrees.
3. Place the chicken breasts on a baking tray and sprinkle with the thyme, salt and pepper. Bake for twenty three minutes.
4. Whilst the chicken is cooking, simmer the broccoli and peas on a low heat.
5. Make the gravy as per the instructions on the packet/tub.
6. Serve and enjoy.

Make time to shop on a Saturday or Sunday (or even better, get it delivered to your door) – this will ensure the fruit you buy will stay fresh until you replenish again on a Wednesday or Thursday for the rest of the week. Also remember, your first shop may look expensive but most of the ingredients such as powdered garlic, sesame oil and soy sauce have many applications and will last you many weeks.

Make sure when you do eat something you know isn't great, write it on your calendar as an amber or red day. This way you can keep track of your 'sins' and keep them as treats you can look forward to by scheduling in a red or amber day. Remember, you can have two amber days or one red day in every seven. Try to keep the red days apart (i.e. don't have one on Sunday and one on Monday) because one day of bad eating when your body is expectant of a low calorie intake shocks your system into a high-metabolic rate which can last into the next day. If you're eating bad on the Sunday, raising your metabolic rate then your low calorie intake on the Monday with your raised metabolic rate will actually help weight loss more than having a low calorie intake for seven days in a row. Your body gets used to a constant low calorie intake to the point where you stop losing weight altogether, in effect, punishing yourself by not eating the foods you enjoy for nothing. Eating badly two days in a row will probably lead to the calories taken in on the second day being stored as fat.

Stage 3 : Managing change

Your resolve, happiness and willpower will be at their strongest on the first day. This may soon be tempered by forcing yourself to eat a high fibre breakfast for the first time and skipping the bacon sandwich you normally have on a Monday morning to help 'kick start' your week. Happiness is paramount to ensuring the transition is a smooth one.

Endorphins are chemicals produced by a gland at the base of the brain during moments of excitement and give us a feeling of well-being. They are thought to be released when we eat spicy food among other activities but just as important is the psychological effect of eating foods we enjoy. The taste, flavour and texture of a food can trigger emotional links to happy moments in your life (such as eating strawberries on a sunny day). Linking flavours with positive emotions is a good way of staying on the right road, especially if your food of choice is a healthy one. As crazy as it sounds, cast your mind back to a happy time and try and pick out a moment when you were eating or drinking something (not alcoholic) you can associate with that moment of contentment.

There are chemical reasons behind why some foods may make you feel happy as well (aphrodisiacs):

Strawberries

They are a good source of potassium which is an important component in the way our nervous system sends messages around the body. If our nerves can communicate more efficiently it reduces the chance of you feeling sluggish and unhappy. Strawberries also contain pelargonidin which is a powerful anti-oxidant.

Pasta

Wholemeal pasta is a source of complex carbohydrate which means it has a low Glycaemic index (does not raise blood sugar quickly) and contains vitamin B, Iron and niacin. Although as yet unproven, there is evidence to support the notion that niacin can help relaxation and treat depression.

Fish

Fish contains GABA (Gamma-amino butyric acid) which is a mood elevator. In medicine, drugs that increase the levels of GABA have relaxing and anti-anxiety effects. Low GABA levels have been associated with headaches, palpitations and depression. The best way to stay happy is to eat foods that can help increase your GABA levels such as bananas, walnuts, broccoli, halibut and fish high in Omega-3 fatty acids such as Tuna and Salmon.

Oranges

Inositol is an almost flavourless carbohydrate found in fruits such as Oranges and Cantaloupe melons. Some studies have shown that taking Inositol supplements can have positive effects on patients suffering from panic disorders and bipolar depression.

Sesame seeds

Threonine is an essential amino acid which the body cannot synthesise and must be taken in through the foods that we eat. Deficiency in threonine has been linked to irritability and negative changes in personality. As well as being high in Omega-3 oils, sesame seeds are a good source of this amino acid, as are eggs, lentils and poultry.

Liver and Kidneys

Phosphatidylserine is a chemical found in offal such as chicken liver and pigs' kidneys. As a sports therapist, I have read many studies which suggest this chemical can accelerate recovery from muscle injuries and even have natural ergogenic (performance enhancing) properties for long distance runners and other sporting pursuits where stamina is required. There is also a school of thought that suggests it can help to enhance a person's mood and relieve stress. As offal is an extremely acquired taste, Phosphatidylserine can also be found in herring, mackerel, tuna, skin-on chicken breast, veal, beef and pork.

Kale

Humans must take in Vitamin B_1 through their diet as it cannot be synthesised. Deficiency of this vitamin can result in malaise (generally feeling unwell), bad temper and confusion. Kale is rich in vitamin B1 (also known as Thiamine), and is also a good source of vitamin K, vitamin C and lutein, which can lower the risk of cataract development. Thiamine can also be found in asparagus, cauliflower, oatmeal and eggs.

Brazil nuts

Selenium is a chemical element which is essential to human biology but only in very small amounts. It plays a role in maintaining correct thyroid function and in the immune system. The amount of selenium in a foodstuff is dependent on the level of selenium in the soil where it was grown. Generally however, Brazil nuts are rich in selenium and other sources include cereal, brown rice and low fat cottage cheese. Some studies suggest that depression , anxiety and fatigue can be caused by selenium deficiency.

Omega-3's

Omega 3 fatty acids are found in fish such as sardines, mackerel and salmon and are believed to play a major role in brain function, especially memory and behavioural functions. As well as many health benefits such as helping the fight against heart disease, high blood pressure and arthritis, deficiency of Omega-3's in the diet has been shown to lead to mood swings and depression. Walnuts are also a good source as they contain a chemical called alpha-linolenic acid which is converted to Omega-3 fatty acids within the body.

The first week

Before you start, draw up a chart on which you can track your progress. You should already know what areas you wish to focus on (such as waist, tummy, thigh and chest girth as well as weight) so make sure the spreadsheet or chart you draw up has boxes for you to write these measurements in each week. If the digital scales you are using also shows percentage body fat and BMI, then make sure you keep track of these too.

- Do you have a pair of jeans or a t-shirt you used to wear but can no longer fit into? This item of clothing is the best way to gauge your progress. Count forward 12 weeks from your start date and write 'try on jeans' on your calendar. There's nothing more motivational than being able to get them past your thighs, and then find you can also get them fastened. Each day you find you've been bad with your diet or a bit naughty – you must move the day you've set to try those jeans on, back one.

- Get your kitchen scales and a sandwich bag. Place the open sandwich bag on the top of the scales and pour some sugar in until the needle reaches the eight ounce mark. Tie this bag off and do the same with another bag until it weighs one pound. I can guarantee there will be a week when you think you've had a great week and find you've only lost half a pound, which will cause you to fling your arms in the air and say 'I don't know why I'm bothering'. What you have to remember is how much your body weight can fluctuate from day to day, but also if you pick up that eight ounce bag of sugar and hold it in your hand, you'll be able to physically see and feel exactly how much weight you've lost – and you'll be surprised how much it actually is. Be proud of yourself.

- Choose a day and time and stick to it. If you've chosen say, a Saturday morning at eight o'clock before breakfast – make sure you weigh yourself every week at that time. It will be even better if you weigh yourself on two consecutive days each week and take an average. If you weigh yourself in between and it seems you've gained weight – just think of how much better you feel both physically and emotionally since you changed your diet.

- Shop twice a week for fresh goods. If you buy a pack of four chicken breasts then place each one in a sandwich bag and freeze it (you can do this with lean pork chops, low fat sausages (two in each bag) and even divide 500g of mince into two 250g bags). That way you can defrost the exact ingredients you need for your meal that evening.

- Make two lists – one of the ingredients you currently have in the house and when one runs out, cross it off the list and transfer it to the shopping list next to it. I can't underline enough how important it is to be organised in the first six to eight weeks of the change in order to make the change a smooth and stress-free one.

- Train yourself to accept the lighter, healthier food choices. Just remember for example how much better for you wholegrain bread is compared to white, regardless of the taste difference.

- Think of the things you do now that you find difficult. Walking upstairs and feeling out of breath or finding it difficult to bend to tie your shoes. Do you get a lot of heartburn? Do you feel bloated after meals? Do you always feel light-headed around eleven o'clock? Make a list of the bad things you feel right now and then dig this list out again eight weeks into your change and see how many you can cross off that list.

- Don't have 'one last take-away'. Start the change right away and don't wait until tomorrow; that's just the old you talking and if you can't start right now, then you're probably not ready for the change and you're still waiting for your 'watershed' moment. If you're tempted to have a take-away, just think how much tastier and better for you the homemade burger is compared to the one about which you have no clue to the ingredients and/or method of preparation from the fast-food restaurant. Remember, you can have that take-away on day seven as your red day as long as you've had six green days. It's probably best to have your red day or amber days on a weekend but if one of your friends is having a mid-week birthday bash or similar, you can go for it without guilt – you'll just need to keep the following weekend green! You'll probably find it easiest to plan your weeks Monday to Sunday but as long as you're only having one red day or two amber days in each seven day period, whichever day you start that period on, then that's fine.

- Remember how important breakfast is. Make sure you have something you're going to enjoy and look forward to in the morning.

- Remember that you're not on a diet; you're changing your lifestyle. Be happy with the choices you've made; try things you've never tried and experiment. Remember you can still eat the foods you enjoy, just adapt them to include good ingredients and reduce your portion sizes.

- Use your calendar every day not just to colour code as green, amber and red. If you had a scoop of fro-yo at the cinema on Friday night (amber), write it down so you know how long it's been since your last treat and what your treat was.

Stage 4 : Up and running

You've done it.

Now that you're up and running, you'll need to *actually* get up and running. The healthiest way to lose weight and maintain your weight loss is to partake in regular physical exercise.

It should be possible to fit exercise into your everyday lifestyle whatever your routine and you don't need to pay expensive gym membership or purchase expensive and cumbersome exercise equipment for your home. Exercise is actually far from the boring and tiring slog that it seems. It's actually a key way of maintaining health and staying happy. As well as triggering natural 'happy' hormones such as dopamine that perk you up, the feeling of satisfaction after you exercise far outweighs the buzz you get from eating a bag of sweets.

Start slow

Whatever method of exercise you choose, make sure you don't do too much too soon and manage your own expectations. If you're not used to exercising, it'll take a while for you to build up to working hard for an entire thirty minutes. Make sure you rest when you feel too tired to carry on and then begin again when you feel able to. If you push yourself too hard at the beginning you can cause all sorts of problem such as strains, sprains and tears to your muscles, tendons and ligaments.

Where to start?

Moderate exercise three times a week should be an achievable and reasonable goal for the first three to four weeks of your new lifestyle. You need to ensure that you keep up a regular routine or any benefit you gain from your last session will be lost if you leave it too long in between sessions. Exercising Monday, Wednesday and Saturday for example is good – doing it Monday, Friday and Saturday isn't as good. However, any exercise is better than none so try to strike a good balance and build up a routine.

What to do?

It will be easier to incorporate exercise into your weekly routine if you enjoy it. Playing physical sports is a great way of getting the exercise you need whatever your ability, but there are several other options available which enable you to exercise at home. There are computer consoles which promote aerobic exercise and many DVD's on the market which contain structured workouts. Be sure to check what equipment you need to carry out the exercises featured on the DVD otherwise you'll get it home and watch eight people rolling around on those big blow-up silver balls whilst standing in front of the television with an exasperated expression. Try sit ups and press ups, keeping a record of how many you managed in your last session. Try to increase the amount next time by one. Not only will this give you motivation, but it's also a good measure of how your fitness is progressing. At the first attempt you may find that the second press up is beyond you. However, soon you'll look at your chart whilst writing the number 20 in today's box to see you could only manage one two weeks ago. It's these small victories that go a long way to changing your outlook on health and fitness. You'll soon be asking yourself the question 'exactly how unfit was I?'

Be sure to drink water during your routine. You will heat up and sweat as you exercise so you need to replace the water you're losing.

What now?

Tailor your workout to the level of fitness you've managed to achieve in the first six to eight weeks. If you're able to exercise continuously for the full thirty minutes whilst feeling moderately out of breath then you have probably reached the level you need to be at to maintain a healthy level of fitness. If you can maintain your exercise at this level then you will be reducing your risk of heart disease among other related conditions. Also, once you have reached this level then three cardio-vascular work-outs per week combined with another two days where you go out for walks or partake in other outdoor pursuits will be sufficient.

So what is it doing?

In terms of weight loss, exercise doesn't do a lot. Exercising alone will have very little impact on your weight. As discussed previously in the book, metabolising fat cells (which is how you lose weight healthily) is your body's call for energy when other sources have been depleted. The body breaks down the fat cells using enzymes which release glycerol and fatty acids into the blood stream. They are then transported to the muscles which then use the fatty acids for energy.

Exercising for half an hour will only burn around 125 calories and unless your blood sugar is extremely low, these calories will not be provided by your fat stores. The key as discussed previously is to change what you eat and use exercise to ensure your body is 'fit' enough to ensure your internal biological processes are efficient. The calories you burn during exercise will use the sugar currently stored in your muscles, which will be replaced by the sugars present in your blood stream. Using blood sugar ensures that any excess isn't converted to and stored as fat. It is the period after exercise that is the most beneficial in terms of weight loss as your metabolic rate has been raised and conversion of blood sugar to fat has been minimised.

Those who exercise regularly often feel that they can 'reward' themselves afterwards with a 'treat'. This defies the point as whatever sugar the treat contains will of course be metabolised more easily, but at the expense of the existing blood sugar. This then nullifies the likelihood of any subsequent internal 'searching' for alternative energy which may have led to your fat stores being raided and used. Eating slow-energy-release foods such as boiled rice and chicken after exercise will ensure your hunger is satisfied for longer and the sugars released into your blood are used and depleted quickly which will send your body off on a search for an alternative source of energy in the form of fat cells.

Remember that 'working' a certain part of your body will not reduce the fat there. If you think you have more fat on your arms than anywhere else, simply using dumbbells to work them out will not mobilise the fat unless you're also controlling your intake of food. Only with regular exercise and the correct diet can you reduce the amount of fat stored in your body and in particular, places where it is more abundant.

When will I see the results?

The reason fad diets are so popular is because they promise results within a short period of time. People who try fad diets rarely educate themselves as to what the diet will do to them physiologically and are not aware that there may be negative side effects. Some people read magazines which show celebrities dropping bottles of diet pills or boasting about how they only drank maple syrup for three weeks and saw dramatic results. These fad diets are not only dangerous and deprive you of the most essential components of your diet, they also cause you to gain more weight than normal when you finally come off them.

It's important to keep in mind, especially for the first four to six weeks, that you might only lose half a pound to a pound a week. The weight loss will not be dramatic as that would be incredibly unhealthy. Remember that you are losing the weight in the right way, in a way that your body can manage and in a way that won't endanger your long-term health. Using the suggestions in this book, it is entirely possible to lose a stone in eight weeks. Take a photograph of yourself from various angles before you start and then again after eight weeks. You'll see such significant changes that you'll be glad you didn't deprive yourself of the foods you love, find yourself fainting at work, grabbing at the stabbing hunger pains as you try to get to sleep and feeling generally unwell for the entire duration of your 'fad diet'. You'll find that the results are significant and you feel so healthy and proud of yourself that the next eight weeks will be easy because it will have become your way of life and you'll forget about the bad old days of takeaway and chocolate.

Don't make excuses

There is a huge difference between allowing yourself a reward using logic and making up a flawed excuse because you are desperate for some chocolate. You'll find that having a treat once or twice a week (such as a scone with Jam on a sunny Sunday afternoon and then having a glass of wine while watching the Wednesday night movie) won't make any difference to your weight loss. You'll still lose weight and you'll still be enjoying the things that you used to eat in much larger quantities and frequency. Your body has everything it needs from your diet and won't panic because of a little extra sugar. If you are dieting using the conventional food depravation method (and therefore sending your body into 'starvation mode'), then the sugar in your scone with jam will be stored as fat much more readily due to your body 'panicking' and preparing itself for whatever emergency it thinks is coming. The types of excuses I have heard dieters make are :

- I didn't have any breakfast so I can have this chocolate bar
- I didn't eat out at the weekend so I can eat whatever I like today
- I don't like what I've brought to work for lunch so I'm going to go to the bakery and get a pasty
- If I leave half of this pizza then I can have ice cream for pudding

Making sure you have three nutritional meals is the key to the whole program. Skipping meals or components of meals doesn't leave a gap for chocolate or any other form of high-fat or high-calorie treat. If you stick to eating correctly and exercising regularly, then a red day or two amber days a week will have negligible impact on your overall weight loss for that week; it might actually help speed it up. As mentioned before, keep a record on your calendar of the treats you've had and compare that with your loss that week; you'll be surprised. Just tailor your eating schedule to ensure your treats (reds and ambers) are exactly that, a 'treat' that you have once in a while and look forward to without guilt.

Conclusion

You have no processed food in the house, only fresh ingredients and low calorie alternatives to the high-flavour high-fat foods you use to have. Slowly but surely you've managed to adapt recipes to your taste by adding the right herbs and spices, using fresh ingredients and realising how lethargic and bloated that other food you used to eat made you feel. You've removed the sins from your diet and replaced them with lower calorie alternatives, gotten used to the taste and don't miss the old stuff. You only have one take away or meal out every week, and realise you don't enjoy it as much as the fresh meals you have been preparing for yourself.

You have the sinful things you weren't able to cut out of your diet in sensible moderation. You're managing your hunger by having healthy snacks such as fruit and hot drinks. You're not demotivated by the relatively slow weight-loss because you know it's being done the correct and healthy way. You're weighing yourself and picking up that half-pound bag of sugar to visualise exactly how much weight you've lost that week and realise it's actually quite a bit so you don't feel downhearted. You're not scared of food; you can have a full Sunday dinner without feeling guilty because you steamed the vegetables, cut the fat off the meat and managed your portion size. You've got more energy because you eat properly at breakfast time and you're eating the correct amounts of vitamins and minerals. When someone offers you a chocolate and you refuse, it's because you're safe in the knowledge that the two grams of saturated fat in the chocolate aren't worth the 'that tastes ok' feeling you'll have for three seconds. In short, you've made a change you can maintain for the rest of your hopefully long and healthy life. If not, then you haven't reached that place in your life which will make you want to change how you live forever.

Also by Peter Nuttall Bsc

No More Stress :

The new technique to manage stress anywhere

No more stress! Based on Pavlov's theories of conditioning you can turn smells and tastes into stress busting 'portable sunshine' in just a few sessions. It's free, you can perform the therapy at home on your own and you don't need any special equipment.

Stress can be managed by practicing relaxation techniques and many people use them to reduce their levels of stress, anger or anxiety.

Total Sense Therapy is not only an ideal at-home, self-administered form of relaxation therapy but also allows you to take that relaxed state of mind with you during the day - a concept known as 'portable sunshine'. When used at home or when you're out and about, Total Sense Therapy can help to decrease stress levels, decrease muscle tension and lower blood pressure among many other potential health benefits. This website is a resource which accompanies the book *No More Stress : the new technique to manage stress anywhere* to help you customise your treatment sessions.